Sciatica Pain
Relief & Posture Exercises

Healing Sciatica and Piriformis Syndrome

Eron Locklear

Contents

Introduction : 4

Anatomy of the Spine in Basic Form: 4

The protrusion, Bulge, and the Herniation of a Disc 5

Rupture / Disc Extrusion 5

Bone and Ligament Thickening Due to Degeneration 6

Piriformis Muscle and Sciatic Nerve 7

Identifying the Source of Your Sciatica 9

The Clues' Interpretation 12

Using Ice And Heat To Relieve Symptoms 13

When in doubt, stay away from the heat! 14

Exercises to Relieve Sciatica Symptoms 15

Exercises based on the McKenzie Method 18

Centralization 19

McKenzie Extension Technique (Advanced) 22

Sciatica Muscle Contraction Exercises 23

Natural Remedies And Supplements 25

Sciatica Prevention : The Importance of Preventative Measures
 29

Lifting And Posture That Is Safe For Your Back 31

Poor Posture When Sitting 31

Proper Sitting Position 32

Position for Sleeping 32

Exercises for Prevention 32

The Pelvic Tilt - The Basic Version: 33

The Pelvic Tilt - The Advanced Version 34

The Slouch and Arch 35

When Should You See A Doctor? 35

Pain Is Turning Into Numbness 37

Introduction :

Symptoms emerging from the sciatic nerve, a big nerve made by multiple smaller nerves branching out from either side of the lower spine, are referred to as sciatica. The sciatic nerves go down the back of each leg, passing through the buttock region on either side. The sciatic nerve separates below the knee into two divisions that run down the leg to the ankle and foot.

Actual sciatica symptoms occur in the buttock region. They may spread down the back of the thigh and into the lower leg and foot, even though some individuals label symptoms elsewhere in the leg sciatica. The more inflamed the nerve, the deeper down the leg the symptoms would spread.

While there are a few neurological illnesses that might produce sciatica owing to direct nerve damage, sciatica is usually a sign of some underlying condition. Nerve compression and muscular contraction are two of the most prevalent causes of sciatica.

Nerve compression may be caused by several things, the most frequent of which is a bulging or rupture of one or more intervertebral discs in the lower lumbar spine.

Anatomy of the Spine in Basic Form:

In normal circumstances, there is plenty of room around the spinal nerves where they branch off from the spinal cord and exit the spine (technically, the spinal cord ends in the mid lumbar spine and becomes a bundle of different nerves called the cauda equina in the lower lumbar, but I'll refer to it as the spinal cord for the sake of simplicity). However, one or more items might limit the aperture where the nerve leaves the spine, causing compression and irritation of the nerve.

A disc bulge, also known as a disc herniation or disc protrusion, is one of the most prevalent nerve compression causes. The discs have an exterior cartilage wall and are filled with a gel-like fluid that allows the spine to move in many directions while absorbing trauma. The gel wall may be damaged (in ways that will be detailed later), causing it to bulge outward at the area of injury due to the internal pressure of the gel. Discs bulge rearward toward the spinal cord and nerves due to the anatomy of the spine and the postures and activities that we regularly participate in.

The protrusion, Bulge, and the Herniation of a Disc

In the extreme instances of disk injury, the disk may rupture, and the inner gel may come thru the disk wall.

Disk rupture or extrusion is the medical term for this.

Rupture / Disc Extrusion

Most disc injuries are bulges or protrusions, which may typically be treated efficiently using the procedures described later in this book. Disc ruptures (extrusions) are more dangerous and often need surgery to provide long-term relief. By the way, the term "ruptured disc" is frequently misused (even by doctors) to describe what is a disc bulge (herniation or protrusion), so don't assume you'll need surgery if you're told you have a ruptured disc until you have confirmation (via an MRI or CT scan) that the disc is ruptured and not simply bulging or protruding.

Changes in the spine caused by degenerative arthritis usually decrease the space surrounding the spinal nerves, in addition to disc bulges and ruptures. Degenerative arthritis causes the discs to lose fluid and grow thinner, the bone surfaces to thicken and develop spurs, and the spinal ligaments to buckle (as the bones get closer together), all of which may constrict the spaces thru which the nerves travel.

Bone and Ligament Thickening Due to Degeneration

Degenerative alterations in the spine often impact the rear side of the spinal apertures, while disc bulges and ruptures typically restrict the front side. There is often some narrowing due to both disc protrusion and degenerative processes. Further nerve compression is usually caused by swelling caused by inflammation produced by disc injury and/or degenerative arthritis.

While tumors and spinal cysts can cause nerve compression and necessitate surgery, most nerve compression cases are caused by a combination of disc bulging, degenerative changes, and/or inflammatory swelling, which can usually be effectively managed with the treatments discussed later in this book.

Muscle contraction is the second most common cause of sciatica symptoms. Although many muscles may produce leg discomfort, only one muscle closely resembles the symptoms of actual sciatic nerve irritation. The piriformis is a muscle that runs from the sacrum (the triangle bone at the base of the spine) to the upper femur, just behind the hip joint, on both sides of the body.

Piriformis Muscle and Sciatic Nerve

The sciatic nerve may run above, below, or straight thru the piriformis muscle, depending on the individual's anatomy. In cases where the nerve passes thru the piriformis, it is thought that muscle contraction or tightness may be enough to cause pressure irritation on the sciatic nerve, but it also appears that the muscle can produce referred pain symptoms that closely resemble the symptom pattern of sciatic nerve irritation. In any case, it's known as "piriformis syndrome," when the piriformis is linked to sciatic nerve complaints.

Piriformis syndrome may be caused by direct muscle damage, such as a fall on the buttocks, although extended durations of sitting more often cause it. Although most instances of piriformis syndrome may be effectively treated with the treatments described later in this book, injections or even surgery may be required to relieve pressure on the sciatic nerve as it travels thru the muscle's core.

It's worth noting that a person may have both piriformis syndrome and nerve compression in their spine at the same time. In reality, since the piriformis muscle is regulated by some of the same nerve components that make up the sciatic nerve, disc bulges, and other compression causes may irritate those nerve components, causing the piriformis muscle to contract excessively and induce symptoms on its own. Some have inferred that ALL instances of sciatica are caused by piriformis contraction as a result of this, but I have not found this to be accurate in my 20 years of clinical practice.

As previously discussed, other muscles might cause sensations similar to sciatica, albeit the symptom pattern is typically unique. Sciatica sensations in the buttock and down the back of the thigh, and sometimes into the lower leg and foot, are caused by nerve compression or piriformis syndrome. Other nerves, muscles, and/or anatomical structures may be involved in symptoms on the side or front of the thigh that is not caused by sciatica or piriformis syndrome. Because there are so many probable reasons for non-sciatic leg pain, this book will treat real sciatica and piriformis syndrome.

As you may expect, since the causes of sciatica differ, the most effective treatment approaches vary as well. As a result, the first step in treating sciatica is to determine the most probable cause(s) and then use the most effective remedies for your specific circumstance.

In the following chapter, you'll learn how to figure out what's causing your sciatica.

Identifying the Source of Your Sciatica

There are various potential causes of sciatica, as outlined in Chapter 1, but most cases fall into one of two categories: nerve compression or muscle contraction.

In certain situations, sophisticated medical testing (MRI, nerve conduction testing, etc.) may be required to identify the exact nature of the issue, and even advanced testing is not always accurate, but the treatments that follow should provide at least some insight into the probable origins of your symptoms.

Keep in mind that each signal is "stand-alone" as we move thru the following hints at the reason for your sciatica. That is, you're seeking a common thread running across the many signs described. For example, if four of the seven indicators point to nerve compression and three are ambiguous, infer the issue is caused by nerve compression.

Take a good posture:
Sciatica caused by nerve compression produced by a bulging disc is often coupled with a lateral displacement of the upper body over the pelvis. However, this is not always the case.

This sort of postural adjustment is the body's unconscious defensive response for reducing pressure on the injured disc. In addition to the sciatica symptoms, there may or may not be lower back discomfort. It is advised not to push oneself straight if you experience this sort of sideways shift since this can exacerbate symptoms. Your posture will gradually return to normal as your health improves.

After a Long Period of Sitting, Get Up :
While both nerve compression due to disc bulging and piriformis syndrome can cause symptoms, when a disc is involved, there will usually be more pain when trying to stand up straight at first, whereas in piriformis syndrome, standing upright does not usually make a significant difference in symptoms.

Symptoms Associated With Heavy Lifting Or Repetitive Bending:
Sciatica that arises within one or two days after performing a lot of heavy lifting or repetitive bending at the waist (like picking weeds) is almost often caused by disc bulging. While most individuals have heard the phrase "lift with your legs," they may not recognize its significance. The mechanical forces on the spinal discs tend to transfer the pressure within the discs rearward as you bend forward at the waist.

Bending forward repeatedly, especially bending forward while lifting anything heavy, puts tension on the rear of the disc wall, causing it to tear or overstretch, resulting in a disc bulge or, in severe instances, a rupture.

Sciatica that appears after a period of inactivity

Sciatica caused by the piriformis muscle is generally connected with inactivity, while disc-related sciatica is associated with bending and lifting. Sitting for lengthy periods without getting up to move about, particularly in someone who is usually more active, may cause piriformis tightness.

Heat-Induced Reaction

Applying a heating pad or soaking in a hot tub is a frequent therapy for any form of musculoskeletal pain. Heat may feel wonderful while being given to nerve compression sciatica caused by a disc bulge or spinal degeneration, but it will typically increase inflammation and worsen symptoms overall in-between applications. Heat, on the other hand, typically eases muscular contraction thus, piriformis syndrome and comparable disorders will generally improve with its application.

The Straight-Leg Test

According to experts, the straight-leg test looks for "nerve root tension," which is an indication of nerve compression and irritation. Simply sit up straight on a sturdy chair and straighten your leg at the knee to do the test.

The Test of the Straight Leg

Even if you only have symptoms in one leg, do this test on both. A rise in discomfort in the affected leg while straightening either leg is a sign of nerve compression, which is most often caused by a bulging disc. During the straight-leg test, symptoms of piriformis syndrome will frequently remain the same or even improve.

Stretching the Piriformis test.

The piriformis stretch test is exactly what it sounds like: it involves stretching the piriformis muscle. To do the test, gently pull your knee toward the shoulder on the other side.

Stretching the Piriformis

Increased discomfort in the buttocks and/or legs is a sign of piriformis tightness, but you should also examine the non-symptomatic leg. Suppose the non-symptomatic limb has increasing symptoms that are roughly the same as the symptomatic leg. In that case, this might be attributable to general inflammation and is not a reliable diagnostic of piriformis syndrome. The increased discomfort may be temporary since the test stretches the piriformis and is both a therapy and a test for piriformis syndrome.

It is both a therapy and a test for piriformis syndrome.

The Clues' Interpretation

As stated at the outset of this chapter, no one sign is dependable in and of itself. You want the majority of the clues to agree on the most probable source of your symptoms out of the seven.

If you don't obtain a clear indication of the probable reason for your condition, I propose that you assume it's nerve compression until an expert assessment proves otherwise. This is because muscular contraction therapies can exacerbate nerve compression symptoms. When you have a muscle contraction issue, you may not get significantly better with nerve compression therapies, but you are unlikely to make the muscle contraction problem worse. So, if in doubt, start with nerve compression therapy.

It's important to remember that nerve compression and muscle contraction may cause symptoms. For the reasons already stated, in such a situation, always start with nerve compression therapies and then go on to piriformis syndrome (muscle contraction) treatments after the severe symptoms have subsided.

With that in mind, let's go on to the following chapter, where we'll talk about how to start treating your pain.

Using Ice And Heat To Relieve Symptoms

One of the most prevalent misunderstandings is when to use ice and when to use heat when it comes to self-treatment. As we covered in the last chapter, ice is more useful when the problem is nerve compression, and heat is more effective when the issue is sciatica caused by muscular contraction. In the last chapter, we explored many clues to determine the origin of your symptoms, but if in doubt, a simple rule of thumb is to decide whether to apply ice or heat based on the symptoms.

If you're experiencing severe or intense pain with or without swelling, inflammation is likely to present, and it's time to apply ice. If your symptoms are simply stiffness or minor discomfort, however, there is typically no significant inflammation present, and heat is a better option in this case.

As a precaution, it's advisable to avoid using heat for at least 48 hours after a trauma or if you suspect you've harmed yourself to ensure that the inflammatory response hasn't been triggered. The inflammation hasn't had enough time to set in.

When in doubt, stay away from the heat!

Although heat feels nice while on (because it improves the transmission of specific nerve impulses that prevent pain signals from reaching the brain), it also raises the body's inflammatory response. When you stop using the heat, you'll notice increased inflammation and discomfort.

Although ice may not provide the same comfort level as heat, it is one of the most effective anti-inflammatory treatments available. The pain of using ice for a short period generally pays off in long-term recovery.

Although some experts advise alternating ice and heat (for example, 10 minutes of ice followed by 10 minutes of heat), I have not found this beneficial. In most cases, picking one or the other depending on the symptoms is typically the easiest strategy. It works just as well, if not better, than attempting to alternate the treatments.

To avoid skin injury, always separate the ice or hot pack from the skin with a layer of fabric, regardless of whether you're using ice or heat. If you wait until the feeling of the analgesic has entirely worn off before applying ice or heat to an area that has recently been treated with Theragesic, Icy Hot, Biofreeze, Ben Gay, or any other topical painkiller; otherwise, the ice or heat might cause skin irritation or injury.

Also, whether using ice or heat, only apply the treatment for approximately 15 minutes, then wait for the skin to recover to an average temperature (about 1 to 2 hours to be safe) before re-applying the therapy. Because the cold or hot feeling may take a few minutes to pass thru the fabric layer between the cold/hot pack and your skin, start timing when you notice a temperature difference on your skin.

Important Note: If you have poor circulation or diminished skin sensitivity due to nerve injury, diabetes, or other factors, see your doctor before using ice or heat.

Exercises to Relieve Sciatica Symptoms

For self-treatment of sciatica, a variety of exercises have been advised. Doctors or physical therapists often offer patients extensive, intricate lists of exercises. Most of these exercises are of little value at best, and most patients don't utilize them for very long due to the intricacy of the workout program.

This chapter will provide you with some workout suggestions that will help you get rid of discomfort as fast as possible. While severe symptoms are present, I recommend using an "intensive care" approach to the exercises, with repeated repetition being the key to symptom reduction.

I want to emphasize the importance of repetition because I've given these recommendations to thousands of people over the years thru my chiropractic office, my websites, and online instructional videos. The importance of frequent repetition in the early stages of treatment is consistently overlooked. This is most likely related to how physicians and physical therapists commonly teach workouts.

Exercises for sciatica are often offered in one of two ways: the patient is either taken through them in a supervised treatment session lasting 15 to 30 minutes, with treatment sessions every day or every other day, or the patient is handed a sheet of exercises and instructed to practice them at home. With these methods, the patient may only complete the exercises once or twice a day. This typically isn't adequate for nerve compression sciatica caused by a bulging disc to provide long-term relief. Thus, patients will frequently be in agony for weeks or months before seeing any improvement.

Always perform a minute or two of efficient workouts numerous times each hour! No, it isn't a mistake; I mean multiple times each hour, not simply once or twice a day.

You may think that's a lot, and you're right, but most individuals don't need to keep up that frequency for very long. In most cases, a few days to a few weeks of using the exercises I'm about to present multiple times per hour will significantly reduce symptoms. Once that happens, you can reduce the frequency of the exercises to just a few minutes per day for prevention (as we'll discuss in the prevention and rehabilitation chapter).

The frequency of the workouts will vary depending on the individual. As a general guideline, for those under the age of 50, I recommend beginning with each exercise for approximately a minute at a time and completing it 5 to 6 times each hour. I recommend starting with a frequency of around half that, at 2 to 3 times per hour, for those over 50. Many older people have spinal arthritis, which might be made momentarily worse by the activities recommended.

During the "intense care" portion of the exercises, many individuals may experience back or shoulder pain. This is generally transient and may be alleviated with the application of ice, as previously mentioned, and/or massage. I suggest continuing with the exercises at the prescribed frequency as long as the discomfort is manageable, but you may permanently reduce the frequency if necessary.

Before I begin the exercises, I'd want to point out that numbness is worse than pain in terms of nerve health.

While most individuals prefer numbness to pain, numbness indicates a higher and/or longer-lasting nerve compression than pain does. So, in most circumstances, if you're beginning with numbness and then moving on to hurt, that's a positive indicator. On the other hand, if you start with significant discomfort and then develop numbness, it's usually a negative indicator that you should stop doing what you're doing and/or get expert help.

So, it's vital to differentiate between numbness, a loss of feeling, and "heaviness" or "tiredness," which may exist after intense pain has passed. If you're not sure, softly poke the affected region with a pin or needle (no need to break the skin) and compare the feeling to the exact location on the other side of your body or another spot that feels normal. If the pin/needle feels the same in both places, the heaviness is likely the effect of muscles relaxing as the nerve irritation subsides.

Let's get started with the pain-relieving exercises..

Exercises based on the McKenzie Method

The McKenzie technique (named after physical therapist Robin McKenzie) is often linked with backward bending of the spine. Still, in truth, it is about identifying and then exercising in postures and stretches that relieve or cause "centralization" of symptoms.

The symptoms become more central as they approach the spine. For example, if you have low back pain and sciatica (leg pain), centralization occurs when the symptoms in the leg fade or disappear, even tho the discomfort in the buttocks or low back remains the same or worsens.

Centralization

In most instances, thigh, buttock, and lower back pain will improve over time after initial centralization has been accomplished.

McKenzie exercises are sometimes referred to as "McKenzie Extension Exercises" since the extension of the spine effectively lowers or centralizes pain the great majority of the time. Still, the real McKenzie Technique checks for the position(s) suitable for an individual patient.

So, although McKenzie exercises often entail spine extension, they may also include flexion (forward bending) and left or right side leaning along with extension or flexion, depending on which posture decreases or centralizes symptoms.

The positions that should be tested and compared to determine the position that best centralizes symptoms are

- Straight Extension
- Extension With Left and Right Side Bending
- Flexion

Note: For flexion, an exercise ball works best, but for testing

For purposes, a pillow or a stack of pillows under the abdomen will work. If

Straight Flexion Is Helpful, Flexion Combined With Left And Right Side

Bending and bending should also be tested, but these positions are rarely used.

And because they can dramatically irritate disc-related symptoms,

These positions are not shown. Again, Flexion With Left and Right Side Bending Should Only Be Tested If Straight Flexion Is Helpful!

When you first start a new job, you will likely experience some discomfort. Observe what changes in your symptoms occur 30 seconds to a minute after getting into each position. It's important to remember that you want to choose a position that initially relieves symptoms furthest away from the spine.

If you have sciatica down to your foot, for example, a helpful position is the one that shifts the pain out of your foot and calf, even if it amplifies discomfort in your buttocks or low back. If you have sciatica in your buttocks and thighs, a helpful posture shifts the hurt out of those areas, even if it worsens the low back pain.

Start with the straight extension position if there isn't a clear "winner" as a posture that best centralizes your symptoms.

Important Note: Avoid any posture that exacerbates symptoms closest to the spine or causes symptoms to spread farther from the spine!

In other words, do not remain in any posture that causes symptoms in the leg to become more acute or to spread farther down the leg.

Important Note: Do not practice any McKenzie exercises if every position creates more significant discomfort at the farthest point from the spine and/or if the symptoms spread farther down the leg from the spine (in such circumstances, professional examination and treatment is highly suggested!).

Otherwise, try experimenting with various positions until you discover one that relieves the symptoms that are the furthest away from the spine the best. Once you've found the optimal position for you, maintain it for 1 to 2 minutes before resting for 30 seconds or so in a neutral posture. Repeat the favorable posture as needed as long as the symptoms closest to the spine are relieved.

Note that you will only use the optimum posture that allows you to centralize the pain.

You will not utilize any of the other positions until the selected posture no longer delivers additional centralization after 3 or more days of regular usage. If this happens, try again to see if an alternative posture is more effective.

One extension postures (straight extension, extension with left side-bending, or extension with right side-bending) will be the most helpful in most circumstances. If this is the case, the following change will generally improve the exercise's benefits.

McKenzie Extension Technique (Advanced)

Start the McKenzie exercise as usual by supporting yourself up on your elbows (and then bend left or right if one of these positions improved your results when using the basic McKenzie extension position).

- Shift your elbows forward an inch or two after that.
- Finally, bring your arms back to pull your upper body back.
- Finally, lift your arms back and forth to drag your upper body forward. Tug strongly enough to feel a pull on the pelvis, but not so hard that your lower body slips.
- This applies moderate traction on the low back, which may be highly helpful when paired with spinal extension.

You may attain comparable results with the spinal extension on your hands and knees as an alternative to resting flat on your back on the floor.

Sciatica Muscle Contraction Exercises

Suppose it looks like nerve compression is causing the majority of your problems. In that case, I suggest skipping the following exercises until your symptoms have greatly improved (unless otherwise advised by a health care professional managing your care). Attempting to stretch muscles that are tense due to nerve compression discomfort may provide little aid until the nerve compression has subsided and, in some instances, can aggravate symptoms momentarily.

As previously said, repetition is crucial to receiving the most significant outcomes, so for the stretches, I'll be discussing, I recommend holding them for 30 seconds to a minute at a time and repeating them 5 to 6 times per hour while you're awake. The frequency guideline is less affected by age than the McKenzie exercises, but you may reduce the frequency as required if you become too sore from practicing the stretches this often.

It's crucial to remember that even if you only feel symptoms on one side, it's still good to complete the exercises on both sides to keep the muscles as balanced as possible. Furthermore, a neurological crossover effect occurs, resulting in greater muscular flexibility on the opposite side of the stretched muscle. Stretching the asymptomatic side will, in some cases, aid the afflicted side. If you're having trouble extending the painful side, try stretching the non-painful side first.

Two muscles typically cause symptoms that are akin to sciatic nerve compression. The piriformis muscle is most often affected. However, the gluteus minimus muscle may also produce comparable symptoms.
Let's have a look at some stretches for these muscles:

Stretching of the Piriformis
The piriformis may be stretched in various ways by flexing (bending forward) and rotating the hip joint inward.

Stretching the Piriformis Muscle
Pull the knee toward the opposite shoulder to stretch the piriformis.
Hold for 10 to 30 seconds before switching to the other leg and stretching it.
Repeat with each leg a few times, and perform the stretch multiple times throughout the day for optimal benefits.

Stretching the Gluteus Minimus
Begin by crossing the ankle of the affected leg across the knee of the opposite leg. Then bring the knee toward your chest from behind; - you should feel discomfort and/or tugging in the buttock region.
Some publications refer to the gluteus minimus stretch described above as a piriformis stretch. While every hip flexion stretches the piriformis to some extent, the hip must be internally rotated to stretch the piriformis to its maximum capacity.

Flexion paired with external rotation stretches the gluteus minimus muscle to its maximum extent.
You may need to extend both muscles to obtain the optimum effects, so if they're both tight, stretch them both and don't worry about which one is which!

That concludes the pain-relieving exercises. In the chapter on prevention, we'll add a few additional exercises, but for now, let's move on to other pain-relieving approaches.

Natural Remedies And Supplements

For sciatica treatment, a variety of nutritional supplements, herbal items, and homeopathic therapies are being pushed. These products are likely to function at least sometimes, whether via a chemical therapeutic action or the placebo effect.

When it comes to sciatica, vitamins and therapies that either has an anti-inflammatory impact or cure some form of nutritional deficit that causes nerve irritation and/or aberrant muscle contraction are more likely to be beneficial.
Because the list of potential supplements and treatments is so extensive, the following suggestions have been restricted to widely accessible supplements and remedies with some level of scientific validation and/or solid anecdotal evidence supporting their usefulness and safety.

The recommendations that follow are for specific vitamins, minerals, herbs, and other supplements, not particular brands. When it comes to brand-name items, you should be aware that marketing hype often outweighs the actual outcomes that may be achieved.

I do not provide particular brand recommendations due to the varying availability of some items in various regions of the globe. When selecting a brand, I suggest looking for one that employs independent lab validation of the product's potency and purity. It's also a good idea to research Amazon.com or another purchasing website to see what other people have to say about the goods.

Anti-Inflammatory Herbs
Anti-inflammatory supplements work by lowering swelling and discomfort by suppressing the inflammatory response. For Omega-3 fatty acids (EPA and DHA – usually from fish oil, but krill oil or walnut oil are other effective sources), bromelain, hesperidin, quercetin, curcumin (turmeric), MSM, ginger, and aloe vera are among the most popular and well-documented by scientific study.

There are various homeopathic medicines for lowering pain and inflammation, and there are many of them. For the most significant outcomes with homeopathy, I suggest visiting a homeopathic physician to find the correct medicine for you.

Natural anti-inflammatories, like medicines, function differently for different people. For simplicity, I suggest taking Omega-3 fatty acids (at a dosage of 1,000 mg EPA per day) or a product that contains a mixture of two or more of the other chemicals indicated (follow package instructions for dosing recommendations). Ginger may be consumed rather than taken as a supplement, and some individuals find candied crystallized ginger to be a delightful and efficient anti-inflammatory. ***

Important Note: If you're already taking anti-inflammatories, whether over-the-counter or prescription or blood thinners like Coumadin (warfarin), you should talk to a pharmacist or licensed healthcare provider before starting any nutritional anti-inflammatories because there could be dangerous interactions.

Getting Rid of Nutrient Deficiencies
A few basic defects may cause sciatica and sciatica-like discomfort.

A lack of any or all of the B vitamins may cause various nerve-related symptoms, such as sciatica. B-6 and B-12 insufficiency are the most frequent B-vitamin deficiencies.

When it comes to vitamin B-6 insufficiency, it's more often than not due to the body's inability to convert the vitamin to the active form known as pyridoxal-5-phosphate (also known as P5P) than a lack of B-6 consumption. As a result, I recommend taking a supplement that includes at least some B-6 in the form of pyridoxal-5-phosphate. I recommend taking 30 to 50 mg of pyridoxal-5-phosphate every day as a dietary supplement.

Vitamin B-12 insufficiency, like vitamin B-6 deficiency, is often caused by circumstances other than regular consumption. To be absorbed and used, vitamin B-12 needs a component created by the body called the "intrinsic factor." In elderly adults and those with a history of alcohol misuse, intrinsic factor production is generally reduced. Because a reduction in intrinsic factors inhibits vitamin B12 from being absorbed, even high oral dosages of B-12 in solid form may not be enough to restore the shortage. In such instances, a deficiency may be treated with either sublingual supplementation or periodic injections of liquid vitamin B-12 by a qualified healthcare professional. Sublingual liquid vitamin B-12 is not as widely accessible as solid supplements. It is not meant to be ingested but instead held in the mouth beneath the tongue for direct absorption into the bloodstream via the mouth's mucous membranes.

Blood testing is highly recommended before beginning either B-12 injections or sublingual supplements to determine whether or not there is a vitamin B-12 deficit. Dosing is determined by the supplement's concentration and the severity of the insufficiency.

Potassium insufficiency is another frequent shortage that may cause sciatica-like sensations. Potassium insufficiency is most frequent in persons who lose a lot of fluid via sweating, vomiting, or diarrhea and those with renal illness. It may also be a side effect of some drugs, particularly diuretics, used to treat high blood pressure.
Mild potassium shortages are generally easily remedied by simply increasing potassium intake in the diet. Although bananas are the traditional high-potassium meal, many other foods are just as excellent, or perhaps better. Melons, avocados, oranges, most green leafy vegetables, and black-strap molasses are among them. Potassium supplements are also available. However, blood testing to determine potassium levels is highly suggested before taking large dosages of potassium supplements - too much potassium may be deadly!

Coenzyme Q-10 deficiency is another deficit that may cause sciatica-like symptoms, albeit commonly as part of all-over body discomfort (or CoQ10 for short). A side effect of cholesterol-lowering medications often causes this deficit. There are two ways to deal with the deficit. The first is to take coenzyme Q-10 supplements at a recommended starting dosage of 200 mg per day. If the symptoms are relieved, the dose may be lowered to 50 to 100 mg per day for maintenance. If there is no benefit and the symptoms seem to be due to cholesterol-lowering medicine, it is suggested that you talk to your doctor about it. You may be able to switch to a different prescription or consider options that would enable you to stop taking it completely.

Although coenzyme Q-10 is typically safe and well accepted, it has the potential to thin the blood, so if you are taking aspirin or a stronger anticoagulant medicine (such as Coumadin), talk to your doctor or pharmacist before beginning it.

Finally, although not strictly a deficit, some people with diabetes may suffer from leg pains similar to sciatica caused by nerve injury caused by poor circulation. Supplementing alpha-lipoic acid, a powerful antioxidant, might occasionally alleviate these symptoms. A daily dose of around 50 mg is advised for long-term usage. For short-term use, higher dosages are sometimes suggested, but only under the guidance of a health care practitioner.

Sciatica Prevention : The Importance of Preventative Measures

It's crucial to remember that the underlying causes of sciatica (particularly bulging discs) usually persist to varying degrees long after the symptoms have faded. It generally only takes a modest decrease in disc bulging and/or inflammatory swelling to minimize or eliminate symptoms. Still, it only takes a minor rise in disc bulging or inflammation for symptoms to return. Even after the symptoms are entirely gone, the underlying bulging disc is generally far from cured. If it is not correctly controlled, it will most likely produce problems again in the future.

Furthermore, although, understandably, patients are shocked when symptoms return after a period of feeling well, it is only logical to assume that the same activities, postures, and lifestyle choices that caused the original episode of sciatica will cause recurrent episodes. This is true for both sciaticas caused by disc compression and sciatica-like symptoms caused by the piriformis and/or gluteus minimus muscles.

With this in mind, I would highly advise folks to think about sciatica management rather than cure. While it would be ideal if there were a cure-all, the fact is that a certain level of continuing preventative treatment is required to avoid the symptoms from reappearing and worsening over time.

Even in many situations when the patient has had surgery, the risk of sciatica recurring is substantial if the patient does not avoid future issues. While a complete discectomy (removal of a disc) ensures that the patient will never have problems with that disc again, such surgeries transfer mechanical pressure to other discs and spinal structures, which often get injured and cause symptoms months or years later. Many surgeons fail to appropriately communicate this to their patients. Thus, these patients are ignorant of the necessity for continuous preventative measures.

The good news is that effective prevention is often simple to implement. While doctors and physical therapists may occasionally give patients a long list of home exercises and other preventive treatments, in my experience, very few patients will continue to spend 20 to 30 minutes or more every day performing a long list of exercises, especially if they are no longer in pain. Fortunately, effective prevention does not require a long list of activities or a lot of time. Doing a few efficient exercises, similar to gaining immediate symptom alleviation, usually works better in the long term than attempting to keep up with various activities.

Most individuals may remain symptom-free for most of the time by combining a few minutes of preventative exercise each day with awareness and avoidance of activities and postures that likely induce sciatica development.

So, let's talk about the most important aspects of avoiding sciatica and other low-back problems.

Lifting And Posture That Is Safe For Your Back

While many people feel that significant pain like sciatica must be caused by a big accident, improper sitting posture (especially when you sit regularly and/or for extended periods) is one of the most common causes of bulging discs, which cause back pain and sciatica.

Poor Posture When Sitting

Sitting with your lower back unsupported puts a lot of strain on the back region of your spinal discs, which may lead to or exacerbate disc bulges that cause sciatica and back discomfort.

When done daily or regularly under even the best of circumstances, prolonged sitting (sitting for more than an hour at a time) may be hazardous to the back. However, keeping an appropriate sitting posture as indicated below will reduce the risk.

Proper Sitting Position

Supporting the lower back when sitting. Even under the best of circumstances, prolonged sitting is stressful on the lower back, so getting up and moving about for at least a minute or two every half hour or so is strongly suggested.

Position for Sleeping

It is worth the effort when sleeping in a "back-friendly" posture might be challenging to achieve (many individuals end up in some quite contorted positions while sleeping).

The ideal sleep positions for most people with back pain and sciatica include laying on their backs with a cushion or folded towel beneath their legs or lying on their sides with a pillow or folded towel between their legs.

Exercises for Prevention

The same activities you performed for symptom alleviation previously should be maintained as a preventative measure but at a lower frequency than during the "intensive care" period.

If your symptoms looked to be caused by a bulging disc and you found relief with one of the McKenzie exercise positions, you should repeat the exercise for a minute or two many times a day. Once you've reached the preventive stage, I suggest doing the matching straight position (extension or flexion) a few times each day if you were utilizing one of the side-bending positions for pain relief (extension with left or right side-bending or flexion with left or right side-bending).

Once you reach the preventative stage, if you had a muscular component and benefited from piriformis and/or gluteus minimus stretching, it is advised that you continue to do those stretches for 30 seconds to a minute a few times on both sides every day.

I recommend that you add a couple of extra exercises to your symptom-relieving activities that target the most frequent weaknesses and imbalances that lead to back pain and sciatica development. The exercises I'm going to give are meant to be acceptable for a broad range of ages and degrees of physical fitness due to the large variety of individuals who are likely to utilize this book. These workouts may be too simple for young, fit people. More strenuous workouts are excellent in such a scenario. Still, it is recommended that you consult with a healthcare expert acquainted with your condition beforehand to ensure that your exercise selection is safe and suitable.

The Pelvic Tilt - The Basic Version:

Begin by laying on your back on a sturdy surface with your legs bent in a basic pelvic tilt.

There should be some room between your low back and the surface you're resting on in this posture (you should be able to slide your hand partway under your low back).

Contract your abdominal muscles and tilt your pelvis so that your low back is pressed on the surface and the gap between your back and the surface is reduced.

Hold the position for around 10 seconds.

Relax and let the space under your back return, then tilt your pelvis the other way for a few minutes to expand the space under your low back.

Return to the starting position by relaxing.

Repeat the complete cycle many times to get acquainted to the movement since the advanced (standing up) version will need a similar action, and it is simpler to gain a feel for the workout while laying down. You may go to the advanced exercise described below if you are comfortable with this form of exercise and can feel the movement in your back and pelvis.

The Pelvic Tilt - The Advanced Version

Start with the Advanced Pelvic Tilt by standing in a comfortable position.

Contract your abdominal muscles, draw them inside, and rotate your pelvis, as demonstrated by the arrows.

Hold for 10 seconds before relaxing.

Relax your abdominal muscles even more, arching your low back slightly and tilting your pelvis.

The pelvis and low back are the only parts of the body that move; the knees do not flex.

In both directions, repeat 10 to 15 times.

If feasible, do this exercise many times every day, as often as possible, if you sit for long periods.

The Slouch and Arch

Starting with the Slouch and Arch, sit on a chair or a sturdy surface with your feet flat on the floor.

If you're sitting in a chair, lean forward slightly so that your back is a few inches from the chair's back.

Allow yourself to hunch with your lower back rounded.

Slowly rise to a very straight posture and maintain it for 10 seconds.

Then, in a steady, controlled movement, let yourself slump again, and after you've reached your slouched posture, begin to sit up straight again.

The slouch and arch exercises move up and down, not leaning forward and backward.

Repeat the exercise, halting just for a moment in the slouch position and maintaining the arch position for approximately 10 seconds each time, alternating between the slouch and arch positions.

One to three sessions per day are typically adequate, with 20 to 25 repetitions per session.

When Should You See A Doctor?

While the focus of this book is on self-treatment, there are situations when professional examination and therapy are required. In most cases, "toughing it out" and giving the body time to recover itself is not a bad idea. However, there are several warning signals to be aware of that suggest the onset of major issues that, if not addressed swiftly, may result in lifelong incapacity.

Cauda Equina Syndrome is a condition in which the cauda equina

Cauda equina syndrome is characterized by acute nerve compression that needs immediate medical intervention to prevent lasting nerve damage. Cauda equina syndrome may include loss of bladder and bowel control, significant paralysis in one or both legs, and "saddle anesthesia," which is a lack of feeling in the inner thighs, lower buttocks, and pelvic region (basically the area that would contact a saddle when horseback riding).

If you acquire these symptoms, you should get medical assistance right away to determine the source and address the problem as fast as possible.

If you don't see any improvement in 2 to 3 weeks, you should see a doctor.

While severe instances might take weeks to heal, and even mild to moderate cases can take weeks to recover completely, a fair rule of thumb is to look for general improvement over any two to three-week period. Most individuals will go thru some ups and downs throughout their recovery, but the trend should be toward improvement over a few weeks. If you haven't already, I highly advise you to contact a doctor if you haven't already done so after 2 to 3 weeks of self-treatment.

Suppose you've previously visited a doctor and aren't getting better. In that case, I suggest asking them to explain any factors that may delay your recovery and give you an estimate of how long it will take for you to start feeling better. If your doctor is unwilling or unable to establish any expectations for you, you should seek a second opinion.

Pain Is Turning Into Numbness

As previously said, numbness is worse than pain from a neurological standpoint, despite being more manageable for most individuals. Numbness is generally a marker of increased nerve compression severity and/or duration and is a sign of decreased nerve function and possibly nerve injury. The longer the numbness lasts, the more likely irreversible nerve damage may develop, making complete recovery impossible.

It's crucial to differentiate between actual numbness (loss of feeling) and the "dull" or "heavy" sensation that might occur when severe pain is removed unexpectedly. If you're unsure, softly poke the region with a pin or needle (don't break the skin!) And compare the feeling to the same place on the other side of the body or a nearby spot that seems normal to you. If the pin/needle poke on the affected location feels substantially less severe, you are certainly experiencing absolute numbness and should seek expert help.

Made in the USA
Middletown, DE
15 February 2025